YOU ARE AMAZING
· REMEMBER · THAT! ·

No act of kindness, no matter how small, is ever wasted

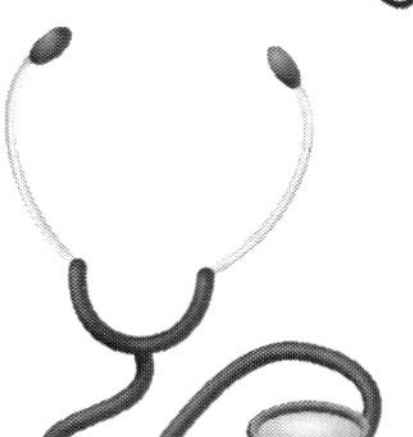

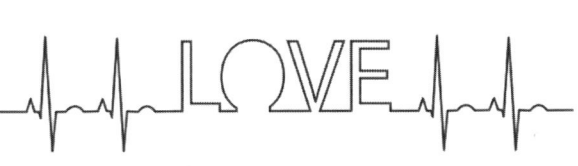

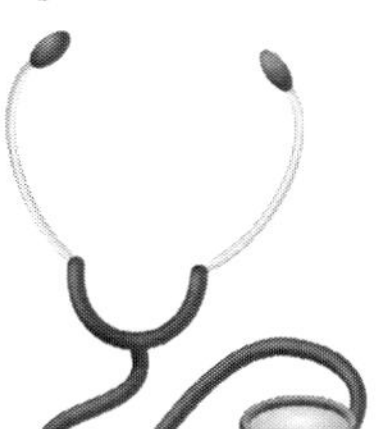

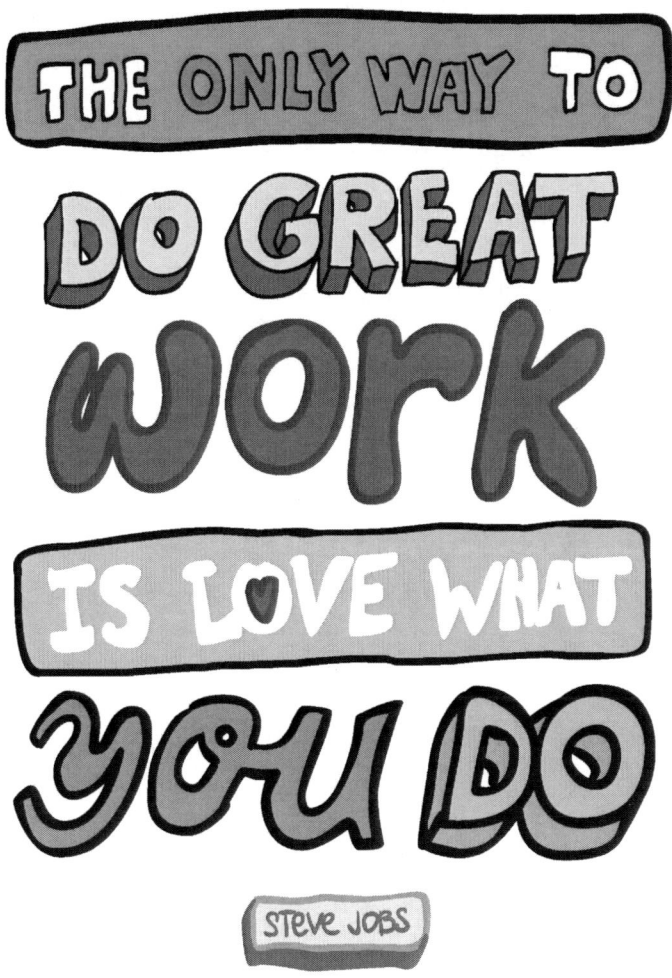

Repeat After Me...

- Today I Will Have Great Compassion & Empathy For The Pain & Suffering of Patients ♥
- Today I Will Have Great Emotional Stability - I Will Not Stress ♥
- Today I Will Have Great Critical Thinking Skills ♥
- Today I Will Have Great Problem Solving Skills ♥
- Today I Will Have Great Time Management Skills ♥
- Today I Will Have Great Communication Skills ♥
- Today I Will Have Great Attention to Detail ♥
- Today I Will Have Great Listening Skills ♥
- Today I Will Have Great Leadership Skills ♥
- Today I Will Have Great Desire To Keep Learning ♥

Nurse Life

When I am in a crisis, I find my hope in my faith.

Nurse Life

○ MONDAY

PRIORITIES

○ TUESDAY

○ WEDNESDAY

TO DO

○ THURSDAY

○ FRIDAY

○ SATURDAY / SUNDAY

MEALS / FOOD

MISCELLANEOUS

ME TIME - READ, WALK, RELAX, SPA, ETC	IMPORTANT STUFF	NOTES/REMINDERS	APPOINTMENTS	GROCERY SHOPPING	LIVE. LOVE. SLEEP. REPEAT.
					M
					T
					W
					T
					F
					S
					S

MONDAY

TUESDAY

WEDNESDAY

THURSDAY

FRIDAY

SATURDAY-SUNDAY

As a nurse, I get better and better every day.

Nurse Life

○ MONDAY

○ TUESDAY

○ WEDNESDAY

○ THURSDAY

○ FRIDAY

○ SATURDAY / SUNDAY

PRIORITIES

TO DO

MEALS / FOOD	ME TIME - READ, WALK, RELAX, SPA, ETC	IMPORTANT STUFF	NOTES/REMINDERS	APPOINTMENTS	GROCERY SHOPPING	LIVE. LOVE. SLEEP. REPEAT.	MONDAY

MONDAY

TUESDAY

WEDNESDAY

THURSDAY

FRIDAY

SATURDAY-SUNDAY

MISCELLANEOUS

M T W T F S S

I will not take other people's negativity personally.

Nurse Life

○ MONDAY

○ TUESDAY

○ WEDNESDAY

○ THURSDAY

○ FRIDAY

○ SATURDAY / SUNDAY

PRIORITIES

TO DO

MEALS / FOOD

MISCELLANEOUS

- ME TIME - READ, WALK, RELAX, SPA, ETC
- IMPORTANT STUFF
- NOTES/REMINDERS
- APPOINTMENTS
- GROCERY SHOPPING
- LIVE. LOVE. SLEEP. REPEAT.

M T W T F S S

MONDAY

TUESDAY

WEDNESDAY

THURSDAY

FRIDAY

SATURDAY-SUNDAY

Whatever I do, I give my best.

Nurse Life

○ MONDAY

PRIORITIES

○ TUESDAY

○ WEDNESDAY

TO DO

○ THURSDAY

○ FRIDAY

○ SATURDAY / SUNDAY

MEALS / FOOD

MISCELLANEOUS

- ME TIME - READ, WALK, RELAX, SPA, ETC
- IMPORTANT STUFF
- NOTES/REMINDERS
- APPOINTMENTS
- GROCERY SHOPPING
- LIVE. LOVE. SLEEP. REPEAT.

M T W T F S S

MONDAY

TUESDAY

WEDNESDAY

THURSDAY

FRIDAY

SATURDAY-SUNDAY

I am an excellent nurse.
Nurse Life

○ MONDAY

○ TUESDAY

○ WEDNESDAY

○ THURSDAY

○ FRIDAY

○ SATURDAY / SUNDAY

PRIORITIES

TO DO

MEALS / FOOD

MISCELLANEOUS

- ME TIME - READ, WALK, RELAX, SPA, ETC
- IMPORTANT STUFF
- NOTES/REMINDERS
- APPOINTMENTS
- GROCERY SHOPPING
- LIVE. LOVE. SLEEP. REPEAT.

M T W T F S S

MONDAY

TUESDAY

WEDNESDAY

THURSDAY

FRIDAY

SATURDAY-SUNDAY

MEALS / FOOD

MISCELLANEOUS

- ME TIME - READ, WALK, RELAX, SPA, ETC
- IMPORTANT STUFF
- NOTES/REMINDERS
- APPOINTMENTS
- GROCERY SHOPPING
- LIVE. LOVE. SLEEP. REPEAT.

M
T
W
T
F
S
S

MONDAY

TUESDAY

WEDNESDAY

THURSDAY

FRIDAY

SATURDAY-SUNDAY

I have helpful co-workers.

Nurse Life

○ MONDAY

○ TUESDAY

○ WEDNESDAY

○ THURSDAY

○ FRIDAY

○ SATURDAY / SUNDAY

PRIORITIES

TO DO

MEALS / FOOD

MISCELLANEOUS

- ME TIME - READ, WALK, RELAX, SPA, ETC
- IMPORTANT STUFF
- NOTES/REMINDERS
- APPOINTMENTS
- GROCERY SHOPPING
- LIVE. LOVE. SLEEP. REPEAT.

M
T
W
T
F
S
S

MONDAY

TUESDAY

WEDNESDAY

THURSDAY

FRIDAY

SATURDAY-SUNDAY

I am grateful for the things I have.
Nurse Life

- ○ MONDAY

- ○ TUESDAY

- ○ WEDNESDAY

- ○ THURSDAY

- ○ FRIDAY

- ○ SATURDAY / SUNDAY

PRIORITIES

TO DO

MEALS / FOOD

MISCELLANEOUS

- ME TIME - READ, WALK, RELAX, SPA, ETC
- IMPORTANT STUFF
- NOTES/REMINDERS
- APPOINTMENTS
- GROCERY SHOPPING
- LIVE. LOVE. SLEEP. REPEAT.

M T W T F S S

MONDAY

TUESDAY

WEDNESDAY

THURSDAY

FRIDAY

SATURDAY-SUNDAY

I am calm and confident.
Nurse Life

○ MONDAY

○ TUESDAY

○ WEDNESDAY

○ THURSDAY

○ FRIDAY

○ SATURDAY / SUNDAY

PRIORITIES

TO DO

MEALS / FOOD

MISCELLANEOUS

- ME TIME - READ, WALK, RELAX, SPA, ETC
- IMPORTANT STUFF
- NOTES/REMINDERS
- APPOINTMENTS
- GROCERY SHOPPING
- LIVE. LOVE. SLEEP. REPEAT.

M T W T F S S

MONDAY

TUESDAY

WEDNESDAY

THURSDAY

FRIDAY

SATURDAY-SUNDAY

My family and friends love me for who I am.

Nurse Life

○ MONDAY

○ TUESDAY

○ WEDNESDAY

○ THURSDAY

○ FRIDAY

○ SATURDAY / SUNDAY

PRIORITIES

TO DO

MEALS / FOOD

MISCELLANEOUS

- ME TIME - READ, WALK, RELAX, SPA, ETC
- IMPORTANT STUFF
- NOTES/REMINDERS
- APPOINTMENTS
- GROCERY SHOPPING
- LIVE. LOVE. SLEEP. REPEAT.

M
T
W
T
F
S
S

MONDAY

TUESDAY

WEDNESDAY

THURSDAY

FRIDAY

SATURDAY-SUNDAY

I will accept nothing but the best.
Nurse Life

○ MONDAY

PRIORITIES

○ TUESDAY

○ WEDNESDAY

TO DO

○ THURSDAY

○ FRIDAY

○ SATURDAY / SUNDAY

MEALS / FOOD

MISCELLANEOUS

- ME TIME - READ, WALK, RELAX, SPA, ETC
- IMPORTANT STUFF
- NOTES/REMINDERS
- APPOINTMENTS
- GROCERY SHOPPING
- LIVE. LOVE. SLEEP. REPEAT.

M
T
W
T
F
S
S

MONDAY

TUESDAY

WEDNESDAY

THURSDAY

FRIDAY

SATURDAY-SUNDAY

I am strong, inside and out.
Nurse Life

○ MONDAY

○ TUESDAY

○ WEDNESDAY

○ THURSDAY

○ FRIDAY

○ SATURDAY / SUNDAY

PRIORITIES

TO DO

MEALS / FOOD

MISCELLANEOUS

ME TIME - READ, WALK, RELAX, SPA, ETC
IMPORTANT STUFF
NOTES/REMINDERS
APPOINTMENTS
GROCERY SHOPPING
LIVE. LOVE. SLEEP. REPEAT.

M
T
W
T
F
S
S

MONDAY

TUESDAY

WEDNESDAY

THURSDAY

FRIDAY

SATURDAY-SUNDAY

I forgive myself for making a mistake.

Nurse Life

○ MONDAY

○ TUESDAY

○ WEDNESDAY

○ THURSDAY

○ FRIDAY

○ SATURDAY / SUNDAY

PRIORITIES

TO DO

MEALS / FOOD

MISCELLANEOUS

- ME TIME - READ, WALK, RELAX, SPA, ETC
- IMPORTANT STUFF
- NOTES/REMINDERS
- APPOINTMENTS
- GROCERY SHOPPING
- LIVE. LOVE. SLEEP. REPEAT.

M
T
W
T
F
S
S

MONDAY

TUESDAY

WEDNESDAY

THURSDAY

FRIDAY

SATURDAY-SUNDAY

ACCEPTED. ACCOUNTABILITY. ALL IS WELL.

Nurse Life

○ MONDAY

○ TUESDAY

○ WEDNESDAY

○ THURSDAY

○ FRIDAY

○ SATURDAY / SUNDAY

PRIORITIES

TO DO

MEALS / FOOD

MISCELLANEOUS

- ME TIME - READ, WALK, RELAX, SPA, ETC
- IMPORTANT STUFF
- NOTES/REMINDERS
- APPOINTMENTS
- GROCERY SHOPPING
- LIVE. LOVE. SLEEP. REPEAT.

M T W T F S S

MONDAY

TUESDAY

WEDNESDAY

THURSDAY

FRIDAY

SATURDAY-SUNDAY

BACKBONE. BALANCED. BOLDNESS.

Nurse Life

○ MONDAY

○ TUESDAY

○ WEDNESDAY

○ THURSDAY

○ FRIDAY

○ SATURDAY / SUNDAY

PRIORITIES

TO DO

MEALS / FOOD

MISCELLANEOUS

- ME TIME - READ, WALK, RELAX, SPA, ETC
- IMPORTANT STUFF
- NOTES/REMINDERS
- APPOINTMENTS
- GROCERY SHOPPING
- LIVE. LOVE. SLEEP. REPEAT.

M
T
W
T
F
S
S

MONDAY

TUESDAY

WEDNESDAY

THURSDAY

FRIDAY

SATURDAY-SUNDAY

CENTERED. CHOSEN. CONSISTENCY.

Nurse Life

○ MONDAY

PRIORITIES

○ TUESDAY

○ WEDNESDAY

TO DO

○ THURSDAY

○ FRIDAY

○ SATURDAY / SUNDAY

MEALS / FOOD

MISCELLANEOUS

- ME TIME - READ, WALK, RELAX, SPA, ETC
- IMPORTANT STUFF
- NOTES/REMINDERS
- APPOINTMENTS
- GROCERY SHOPPING
- LIVE. LOVE. SLEEP. REPEAT.

	M
	T
	W
	T
	F
	S
	S

MONDAY

TUESDAY

WEDNESDAY

THURSDAY

FRIDAY

SATURDAY-SUNDAY

I am thankful for being who I am.
Nurse Life

○ MONDAY

PRIORITIES

○ TUESDAY

○ WEDNESDAY

TO DO

○ THURSDAY

○ FRIDAY

○ SATURDAY / SUNDAY

MEALS / FOOD

MISCELLANEOUS

- ME TIME - READ, WALK, RELAX, SPA, ETC
- IMPORTANT STUFF
- NOTES/REMINDERS
- APPOINTMENTS
- GROCERY SHOPPING
- LIVE. LOVE. SLEEP. REPEAT.

M
T
W
T
F
S
S

MONDAY

TUESDAY

WEDNESDAY

THURSDAY

FRIDAY

SATURDAY-SUNDAY

I take pleasure in my life.

Nurse Life

○ MONDAY

PRIORITIES

○ TUESDAY

○ WEDNESDAY

TO DO

○ THURSDAY

○ FRIDAY

○ SATURDAY / SUNDAY

MEALS / FOOD

MISCELLANEOUS

- ME TIME - READ, WALK, RELAX, SPA, ETC
- IMPORTANT STUFF
- NOTES/REMINDERS
- APPOINTMENTS
- GROCERY SHOPPING
- LIVE. LOVE. SLEEP. REPEAT.

M	
T	
W	
T	
F	
S	
S	

MONDAY

TUESDAY

WEDNESDAY

THURSDAY

FRIDAY

SATURDAY-SUNDAY

MEALS / FOOD

MISCELLANEOUS

ME TIME - READ, WALK, RELAX, SPA, ETC	IMPORTANT STUFF	NOTES/REMINDERS	APPOINTMENTS	GROCERY SHOPPING	LIVE. LOVE. SLEEP. REPEAT.
					M
					T
					W
					T
					F
					S
					S

MONDAY

TUESDAY

WEDNESDAY

THURSDAY

FRIDAY

SATURDAY-SUNDAY

I WIN at everything I do. Failure is not an option.

Nurse Life

○ MONDAY

○ TUESDAY

○ WEDNESDAY

○ THURSDAY

○ FRIDAY

○ SATURDAY / SUNDAY

PRIORITIES

TO DO

MEALS / FOOD

MISCELLANEOUS

ME TIME - READ, WALK, RELAX, SPA, ETC	IMPORTANT STUFF	NOTES/REMINDERS	APPOINTMENTS	GROCERY SHOPPING	LIVE. LOVE. SLEEP. REPEAT.
					M
					T
					W
					T
					F
					S
					S

MONDAY

TUESDAY

WEDNESDAY

THURSDAY

FRIDAY

SATURDAY-SUNDAY

DEPENDABLE. DETERMINE. DEVOTED.

Nurse Life

- ○ MONDAY

- ○ TUESDAY

- ○ WEDNESDAY

- ○ THURSDAY

- ○ FRIDAY

- ○ SATURDAY / SUNDAY

PRIORITIES

TO DO

MEALS / FOOD

MISCELLANEOUS

- ME TIME - READ, WALK, RELAX, SPA, ETC
- IMPORTANT STUFF
- NOTES/REMINDERS
- APPOINTMENTS
- GROCERY SHOPPING
- LIVE. LOVE. SLEEP. REPEAT.

					M
					T
					W
					T
					F
					S
					S

MONDAY

TUESDAY

WEDNESDAY

THURSDAY

FRIDAY

SATURDAY-SUNDAY

EASY TO TALK TO. ENTHUSIASM. EXCEPTIONAL.
Nurse Life

○ MONDAY

○ TUESDAY

○ WEDNESDAY

○ THURSDAY

○ FRIDAY

○ SATURDAY / SUNDAY

PRIORITIES

TO DO

MEALS / FOOD

MISCELLANEOUS

- ME TIME - READ, WALK, RELAX, SPA, ETC
- IMPORTANT STUFF
- NOTES/REMINDERS
- APPOINTMENTS
- GROCERY SHOPPING
- LIVE. LOVE. SLEEP. REPEAT.

	M
	T
	W
	T
	F
	S
	S

MONDAY

TUESDAY

WEDNESDAY

THURSDAY

FRIDAY

SATURDAY-SUNDAY

I support others with love and kindness.

Nurse Life

- ○ MONDAY

- ○ TUESDAY

- ○ WEDNESDAY

- ○ THURSDAY

- ○ FRIDAY

- ○ SATURDAY / SUNDAY

PRIORITIES

TO DO

MEALS / FOOD

MISCELLANEOUS

- ME TIME - READ, WALK, RELAX, SPA, ETC
- IMPORTANT STUFF
- NOTES/REMINDERS
- APPOINTMENTS
- GROCERY SHOPPING
- LIVE. LOVE. SLEEP. REPEAT.

	M
	T
	W
	T
	F
	S
	S

MONDAY

TUESDAY

WEDNESDAY

THURSDAY

FRIDAY

SATURDAY-SUNDAY

I am proud myself.
Nurse Life

○ MONDAY

○ TUESDAY

○ WEDNESDAY

○ THURSDAY

○ FRIDAY

○ SATURDAY / SUNDAY

PRIORITIES

TO DO

MEALS / FOOD

MISCELLANEOUS

- ME TIME - READ, WALK, RELAX, SPA, ETC
- IMPORTANT STUFF
- NOTES/REMINDERS
- APPOINTMENTS
- GROCERY SHOPPING
- LIVE. LOVE. SLEEP. REPEAT.

M
T
W
T
F
S
S

MONDAY

TUESDAY

WEDNESDAY

THURSDAY

FRIDAY

SATURDAY-SUNDAY

I am excited of the unknown.

Nurse Life

○ MONDAY

○ TUESDAY

○ WEDNESDAY

○ THURSDAY

○ FRIDAY

○ SATURDAY / SUNDAY

PRIORITIES

TO DO

MEALS / FOOD

MISCELLANEOUS

- ME TIME - READ, WALK, RELAX, SPA, ETC
- IMPORTANT STUFF
- NOTES/REMINDERS
- APPOINTMENTS
- GROCERY SHOPPING
- LIVE. LOVE. SLEEP. REPEAT.

M T W T F S S

MONDAY

TUESDAY

WEDNESDAY

THURSDAY

FRIDAY

SATURDAY-SUNDAY

FABULOUS. FLEXIBLE. FORTUNE.
Nurse Life

○ MONDAY

PRIORITIES

○ TUESDAY

○ WEDNESDAY

TO DO

○ THURSDAY

○ FRIDAY

○ SATURDAY / SUNDAY

MEALS / FOOD

MISCELLANEOUS

- ME TIME - READ, WALK, RELAX, SPA, ETC
- IMPORTANT STUFF
- NOTES/REMINDERS
- APPOINTMENTS
- GROCERY SHOPPING
- LIVE. LOVE. SLEEP. REPEAT.

	M
	T
	W
	T
	F
	S
	S

MONDAY

TUESDAY

WEDNESDAY

THURSDAY

FRIDAY

SATURDAY-SUNDAY

GAME-CHANGER. GOOD SAMARITAN. GOODHEARTED.
Nurse Life

○ MONDAY

○ TUESDAY

○ WEDNESDAY

○ THURSDAY

○ FRIDAY

○ SATURDAY / SUNDAY

PRIORITIES

TO DO

MEALS / FOOD

MISCELLANEOUS

- ME TIME - READ, WALK, RELAX, SPA, ETC
- IMPORTANT STUFF
- NOTES/REMINDERS
- APPOINTMENTS
- GROCERY SHOPPING
- LIVE. LOVE. SLEEP. REPEAT.

					M
					T
					W
					T
					F
					S
					S

MONDAY

TUESDAY

WEDNESDAY

THURSDAY

FRIDAY

SATURDAY-SUNDAY

HAPPY-GO-LUCKY. HARD WORKER. HEALING.

Nurse Life

○ MONDAY

PRIORITIES

○ TUESDAY

○ WEDNESDAY

TO DO

○ THURSDAY

○ FRIDAY

○ SATURDAY / SUNDAY

Manufactured by Amazon.ca
Acheson, AB